Sensual M Beginners:

Complete Guide on Sensual Massage, Rules, Techniques, Gains, Steps & Many More

By

Dr. Malik J. Dahlberg

Copyright@2023

TABLE OF CONTENTS

CHAPTER 1

INTRODUCTION

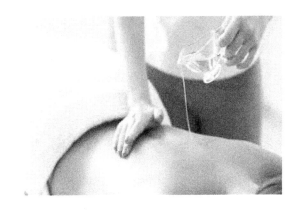

Sensual Massage Meaning

Sensual massage involves stimulating
a partner's touch with hands and
body. It is regarded as a healthy
technique to improve a couple's
sexual intimacy by relaxing and

exciting both members. Benefits include increased intimacy and lovemaking.

Sensual massage begins with a conventional body massage and then gently focuses on the client's privates. Private portions are privaties. It will be a gentle therapy with rich aroma and strong sexual soundtrack to make the customer feel happy. After the usual body massage, the masseuse gently focuses on the vaginal and nipples, arousing and hardening them to get the feeling. Adding lubrication to the clitoris as well as shaking it gives a sexual experience. Also, nipples are softened and made erect. After massaging nipples, breast, and clitoris in one go, the speed increases and when the client is satisfied putting the fingues into her vagina, she gets fingered. That will be done swiftly. There's no rush. Sensual massage involves serene, gentle massage till the customer is satisfied. Breast and nipple massage usually relax women, as does clitoris hood massage.

Some trigger points are held and massaged in all massages to make the client feel good. The client must lie horizontally with her chest looking downwards so the massage can begin at the back. Focusing on her ass. After flipping the client, the front side is massaged. Focusing on privatization. Usually an hour or 90 minutes. It's time-consuming, but clients feel differently because it's different.

History

Sensual massage has a long history. Chinese and Indian cultures used this touch 1,500 – 2,000 years ago. India pioneered sensual massages like tantric massage that combined spirituality and physicality. Modern couples are reintroducing massage as a sexual activity in the West, where it was traditionally employed for healing.

CHAPTER 2

THE TOOLS AS WELL AS TECHNIQUES PLUS AMAZING TIPS

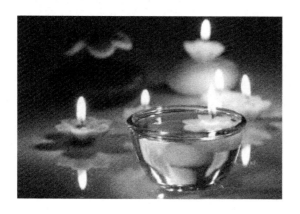

Tools

Tools for sensual massage provide for a wide variety of sensory experiences. When massaging, many people prefer to use massage oils or lotions. Some of these have aromas that calm or energize the receiver, while others, like almond oil, simply assist the massage therapist's hands glide over the receiver's body without causing any friction. Some masseurs will use textured objects to heighten the gratification of a sensual massage. Feathers and other fabrics like silk and velvet are examples.

Techniques

Sensual massage can involve a variety of approaches. The fan stroke, the circle stroke, and the stretching stroke are some of the most common. In order to calm and relax the receiver, a sensual massage typically begins with gentler stroke variations before progressing to firmer or harder techniques later in the massage.

Implications for Physiology

The physical consequences of a sensual massage are an integral component of the overall experience. A sensual massage can improve circulation all over. Further, it raises levels of the feel-good hormone oxytocin and lowers those of the stress hormone cortisol. Regular massage can also contribute to increased immune function and greater general health overall.

Ways to Give Your Partner the Best Massage

Whether in a spa or relaxing on your couch, receiving an excellent massage can be euphoric. If you want to improve your amateur masseuse abilities for a loved one I have some great advice for you. These are explained below:

i. Their Face

Press your partner's temples gently with two fingers coming from each hand for several seconds. Then, carefully stroke their cheeks in little circles as you inch downwards their face. Once you approach the jaw, gently trace their lips using the index finger. Sensory neurons on the lips' outside edge cause significant pleasure.

ii. Their Neck Front

Caressing here activates the thyroid, a small neck gland that controls energy and sex. Trace circles around the Adam's apple using your fingertip in wide, flowing motions. Next, sweep your lips around the throat hollow and massage it with your tongue in wide, soft circles.

iii. The Ear

Gently grip and tug the earlobe between the thumb and forefinger while tracing the C-shaped region on his outer ear with your tongue. Start mild and slow if it tickles.

iv. The Lower Back

Acupuncturists think the kidneys in the lower back above the waist provide sexual vitality. Find the sacrum, a flat triangle bone between his hips at the bottom of the spine. The sacrum has tiny nerve-filled openings. Knead it to warm the skin with your palms. Trace your fingertips upward from the spine base with firm pressure.

v. The Palms

Try gently massaging your inside palm. Feels great, right? Circle your partner's outside palm with your fingertips and slowly move to the middle, the most sensitive spot. The wait is worth it.

Bonus stroke: Slide your fingertip over the pinkie's edge where it joins his hand.

vi. The Stomach

Tap two fingertips from naval to penis base slowly. Next, use your fingertips to circle his belly button, getting larger as you approach his outside abdomen. Adjust speed and apply pressure so as to prevent

tickling him. You want moans, not
laughs.

vii. Behind the Knees

The skin below the knees is thin and
full of sensitive nerve endings. Lay
your partner on his stomach and
softly scratch under each knee to
heat the area before sliding your
tongue in loops across the crack.

viii. The Ankle Dip

A finger-tip-sized, unnamed pressure
point between the heel as well as
ankle bone feels heated when
stimulated. Two fingers should slide

from the ankle bone to the hollow indentation over his heel. Continuously pulse your fingertips into the indent. Lightly lick the region up-and-down to change the sensation.

A straight line connects the foot to other erogenous areas. Take your fingertips from the bottom of his heel to his foot pad below his toes. Rub the pad circularly with your thumbs. Press hard to avoid tickling. Bring the big toe towards you and kiss or suck it for an extra sensual surge.

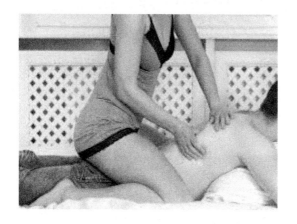

CHAPTER 3

SENSUAL MASSAGE BENEFITS

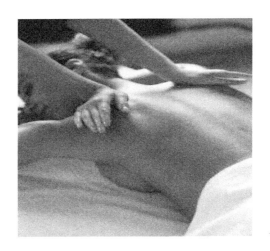

Erosive massage has numerous as well as surprising health benefits

Besides great pleasure in excitation and sexual connection, a sensual massage provides unparalleled relaxation and nurtures your body and spirit. Erotic stimulation and orgasm have numerous unnoticed health benefits. Here are eight unexpected ways that a sensual massage might improve your health.

i. Immune system booster

Regular treatment with massage has long been shown to enhance white blood cells, that fight disease. Add sensuous elements to the service and the benefits grow. Regular intercourse has been shown to increase an antibody that fights germs and viruses. Erotic massages reduce sick days.

ii. As exercise

How often does one promise to get active but never do? Erotic massages are workout. A 45-minute massage burns slightly under 70 calories, according to modern research. Electrifying passion, taking control, and shifting positions can significantly amp up your session calories. Wild sex burns 120 calories. Who needs a treadmill when a gorgeous oriental masseuse can get you sweaty?

iii. Reduces heart attack risk

Good sex is said to be the secret to a healthy heart, and it's true! A bump 'n' grind raises your heart rate and regulates estrogen and testosterone. Low hormones can cause many issues. Osteoporosis and heart disease are examples. Men who have sex at least multiple times a week are twice as likely not to pass away of heart disease, according to research.

Erotic massage can help you keep your heart healthy!

iv. Reduces pain

Are you tired of using massive amounts of ibuprofen and paracetamol to relieve your pain? Erotic massages can replace painkillers. A beautiful oriental therapist releases endorphins. By blocking signals that cause pain from reaching the brain, endorphins are called natural painkillers. Erotic massages relieve headaches, backaches, and more.

v. Reduces prostate cancer risk

Research indicated that men with regular experiences are less probable to have prostate cancer. Although several variables increase cancer risk, regular sensual massage therapy won't hurt.

vi. Relief from sleep issues

If you have insomnia, an erotic massage may help. A skilled oriental therapist boosts serotonin, a hormone essential for sleep. The strokes also soothe the body as well as mind and remove bad ideas, which helps people sleep more!

vii. Increases sexual endurance

Practice makes perfect, and sexual massage therapy gives you stallion stamina. Erotic massages teach you what you like and how to maximize intimacy. If you want to impress your lover while offering them a memorable night, a massage with erotica is the perfect rehearsal!

viii. Reduces stress

Naturally, a massage relieves tension, but adding eroticism boosts the benefits. Massage alone breaks down adhesions (muscle knots) and eliminates cortisol, providing the most relaxation. Erotic massages relieve stress physically and emotionally. A joyful ending produces Oxycontin, which boosts pleasure and positivity. Those who experience regular orgasms are twice as happy. Erotic massages are the ultimate stress alleviation.

CHAPTER 4

SENSUAL MASSAGE DOS AND DON'TS

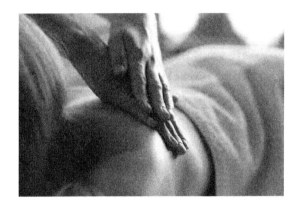

How often have you massaged your
lover for more than a few mins of
shoulder pressing while watching TV
or a half-hearted palm swish?

Anything more makes your thumbs throb or back hurt.

i. Don't spray your partner with oil. Splashing cold oil on warm skin feels awful in real life but looks lovely in movies. Squirt oil into a single hand and rub between your palms to warm it before spreading to the body.

ii. Speaking of oil, avoid body creams because they soak fast and disrupt massage flow. The best oil is sweet almond or apricot if your companion is allergic to nuts. These mild, readily absorbed oils are perfect for massage because they won't harm towels, linens, or clothing (they wash off easily). Using a soft towel to wipe off excess oil from your spouse can be part of the massage, continuing your massage strokes.

Iii. Slow down. Lots of couples speed through their massage. No points are awarded for completing first, and you don't need to start deep and firm (unless your partner wants a leg rub stat after football). Gentle strokes soothe your spouse and warm up the muscles. The slowed down will also build trust, making them willing to cooperate by the end. You dive deep then.

iv. Don't thumb! Not initially. Avoid using thumbs until the massage is over because they fatigue hands quickly. Use an open-hand method with relaxation strokes for 10 minutes, then use your thumbs for brief strokes on certain knots.

v. Request feedback. You should ask for client comments like any professional massage therapist. "Is that far down enough?" "How does this location feel?" and so on are good inquiries. While massaging, check for moans, groans, and oohs and aahs; they indicate good work. If

you get a massage, give positive
reviews. Positive reinforcement is
key: tell your partner how fantastic
the massage feels and let out a few
discreet oohs and aahs. Criticism will
demotivate them.

vi. When receiving, don't expect a
massage. Expectations cause most
fights, right? Expecting a massage is
impolite. You should massage your
lover to do something pleasant for
them and say so before you start. If
they're decent, they'll support you
another night.

vii. Prepare before massaging. Turning off lights, answering the phone, or getting a towel mid-massage is not ideal. Start with everything arranged and nearby. Turn off your cell phone!

viii. Fit the hands that belong to your companion. Massages feel better with greater surface area touched. For massage, keep fingertips as well as palms lowered and relaxed. Tense hands won't contour well and won't feel natural during massage.

ix. Don't underestimate atmosphere. Keep the massage environment clean and enticing by lighting candles, playing soothing music, burning incense (if your partner likes it), and serving wine and chocolate.

x. Massage along the floor without lying down. The bed seems seductive, but the soft, uneven mattress will harm your back and your partner's neck, making it impossible to relax. Kneeling on the ground with another person cross-legged is preferable. Cushion your butt to reduce knee stress. Such a posture gives you good access to your partner's neck, shoulders, arms, as well as upper back. You should massage for a maximum of twenty minutes in that position because it will exhaust your knees as well as lower back. Despite popular assumption, lying down for massages is not sexier or just more comfortable for both of them.

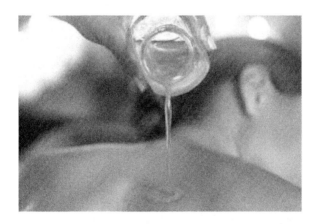

CHAPTER 5

SEXUAL THERAPEUTIC MASSAGES THAT WILL LEAVE YOUR PARTNER LUSTFUL

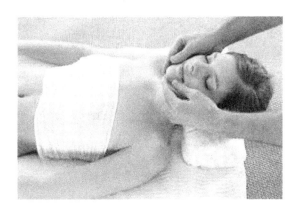

Many massages exist, but sensual massages are most significant. Sexual massages relieve body tension and stress, improving the recipient's well-being. Erotic massages don't always aim to climax or ejaculate, but they can help people focus on the pleasure.

As you discover each other's bodies, erotic massage can strengthen relationships. Massages can also treat health-related sexual pains, release sexual muscles for penetration or orgasm, relieve daily stress, help someone fall asleep, and relieve headache discomfort.

Sexual Massages for Your Partner

i. Two- or Four-Hand Massage

The Duo or just Four Hands Massage involves two people lavishly massaging the recipient's entire body. Masseuses rub massage oil on themselves and the recipient.

Body-to-body massages usually follow this form of therapy. While watching two people therapy their body, the Duo Therapy can be overwhelming.

ii. Nuru (body-to-body) massage

The Nuru or Body-to-Body Massage begins with the masseuse undressing. They apply massage oil to customers and themselves. The massage oil is tasteless and odorless. Masseuses then rub their bodies on customers.

Nuru denotes "slippery" in Japanese. The Nuru Massage may lead to sexual activity according to the person.

iii. Lingam/Penis Massage

The Lingam or just Penis Massage
signifies "Wand of Light." Male penis
is the wand of light. The masseur
honors penis sensations and
stimulation with the Lingam Massage.
The shaft, the testicles, perineum, as
well as external prostate are
massaged.

This sort of sexual massage aims to
give you all the benefits of a genital
massage! Ejaculating is optional, but
they don't mind. Man receiving
massage will learn to enjoy it.

iv. Yoni/Vagina Massage

Yoni, or vagina massage, honors, loves, and respects the vagina's natural stimulation. The Sanskrit word Yoni signifies sacred space or just temple. Start a Yoni Massage in a relaxed state to experience and embrace the pleasure.

This sort of sensual massage also involves the giver loving the massage to create trust and respect. Women utilize this massage to relieve sexual problems like anorgasmia and discomfort. Similar to the Lingam Massage therapy, the Yoni Massage aims to make the recipient enjoy the procedure, not orgasm.

v. The Tantric Massage

The Tantric Massage has Indian yoga plus sex therapy roots. Tantra, the "science of ecstasy," involves giving and receiving sexual awareness and spirituality.

The recipient just thinks about the experiences as well as their well-being. Tantra encourages rest, not orgasm.

vi. Prostate Massage

Male prostate gland stimulation is provided by prostate massage. Tantra calls the prostate a man's emotional, sexual, and holy region. Prostate stimulation releases both mental and physical pressure. A slow external prostate stimulation of the perineum leads to gradual anus stretching.

A lover or partner can massage the prostate, a strong experience. A Lingam Massage is typically added to a Prostate Massage for extra pleasure.

vii. Soap Massage

The Soapy Massage involves two or more persons in a shower. One or all are naked. The giver lathers or massages soap onto the body. A Soapy Massage clears them for sex or massage.

viii. Happy End Massage

Happy Ending Massages directly stimulate the genitals to induce orgasm. A joyful conclusion is called a hand operation and might last a long time.

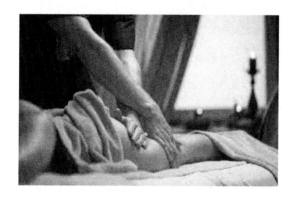

CHAPTER 6

STEPS TO GIVE YOUR SPOUSE AN EROTIC MASSAGE

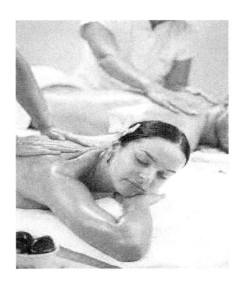

The correct items and methods to turn on and relax your mate

Want to provide your lover a sensuous, relaxing massage? Steamy massages are fantastic foreplay and a great way to demonstrate to your lover you appreciate them. My advice will help you deliver a great massage even if you're not a pro. Read on to give your partner a memorable massage.

You Should Know

Dim the lighting and burn incense to prepare for the massage.

Undress with your spouse to render the massage experience more sensual and pleasant.

Massage your partner's neck, shoulder blades, and legs with massage oil or lotion.

i. Set up an environment with candles as well as incense

Dim the lighting and use soothing music to relax your companion.

Dim the lighting and use soothing music to relax your companion. You could give your lover the nicest massage in the entire globe, but the lighting and music may not be comfortable. Invite your spouse to lie down with candles, incense, and seductive music.

Since your lover is already lying in a soft, comfortable bed, giving an oil massage in his or her bedroom is easy. Before starting, lay down some towels to avoid oil on your sheets.

Relaxing essential oils like lavender or just bergamot can be diffused.

ii. Undress with your spouse

Make the massage experience more intimate by massaging naked.

You're not offering a professional massage, so don't be professional. Ask the other person to take themselves down, subsequently do the same—it will make the massage more fun and pleasant.

Wear a robe with a unique feature underneath to avoid stripping. New lingerie or underwear will delight your lover.

iii. Apply lotion or just massage oil

Lotion...

Your hands glide over your partner's body with lotion or oil. Without oil, you can perform a decent massage, but your partner will lose out. Heat a massage oil or lotion you both like in both hands before starting.

Buy high-quality massage oils since they absorb into the skin. Good oils include jojoba and almond. Despite appearances, food oils including olive, coconut, or just cocoa butter can be effective massage oils. Many masseurs choose basic oil for cooking on the skin.

You can also prepare massage oil by soaking calendula, lavender, the rosemary plant or just other aromatic herbs or oils that are essential in natural oil.

iv. Shoulders and back of neck first

Start massaging the shoulders and neck, which are very tense.

Use your thumbs to softly slide down the vertebral column on the lower part of the neck. Work little circles along the sides of the neck, watching your partner's reaction.

Another good site to hit is where your neck joins your shoulder, paying attention to the shoulder blade. Always follow the bone, not cross it.

Another good spot to massage is the bottom of the head, where tension is high. Gently work that area using your fingers and thumb without over-pressing.

v. Palm pressure should be firm and even

Your palms relieve tension and muscle strains.

Massage methods differ, but there's no secret about how to make your lover feel wonderful. Gently rub your partner's muscles with lengthy strokes. Push with the bottom of your palm and reach for sensitive regions with other portions of your hand.

Instead of pushing on bones, massage muscles. It feels wonderful when you stroke the inside of someone's forearm, but not pushing hard on their elbow.

Thumb massage is possible, but sparingly. Save thumbs for major, stiff muscles like legs, glutes, and shoulders.

vi. Massage the lower part of the legs

To relax your partner's legs, release tension.

Paying particular regard to the calves, massage both large back leg muscles separately. An excellent massage can depend on this. For sore spots, work using the thumbs up along with both back thigh tendons.

Don't be hesitant to touch your partner's sensitive crotch as you come closer. Avoid sex before a proper massage—it takes time!

vii. Treat your lover to foot massage

Massage your partner's feet head-to-toe.

Slide a thumb along your partner's foot arch for a romantic foot massage. Apply oil freely to each toe then utilize both thumbs to make small circles on the foot region. Apply strong pressure to the foot to avoid tickling.

If you always massage head-to-toe, try something new. Work up from the feet.

viii. Focus on neglected bodily parts

Remember your hands, ears, as well as knees! Everyone knows touching genitals along with other erogenous areas feels fantastic. Going straight to these places can result in a rushed or crude massage. Be patient and explore neglected body parts for the most sensual and meticulous massage as long as your spouse is comfortable (communicate!). Do not overlook:

The wrists

The foot arch

Fingers and palms

The back of neck

The ears

Behind the knees

ix. Try full-body strokes

Go over your partner again to relax
their muscles.

After applying lots of oil to your partner's body, make long, full-body sweeps with your palms. Revisit all the massaged areas slowly. This might make a lovely massage ending. It may additionally feel pleasant to massage your forearm or knuckles differently from before.

x. Consult your partner for advice

Let your spouse tell you what seems good and bad.

Not sure what to start a massage
next? Ask your lover where they hurt.
This will indicate where to go and
what to prioritize.

Ask "Is it also firm?" or "Does it seem
good?" when moving to a new body
part. Pay attention and adapt your
massage.

xi. Be patient

Slowly massage your partner's entire
body.

Not every massage leads to sex. Let the massage last, treating your companion to sensual touches since they feel beneficial but not because they could give rise to more. Slower massages allow you to feel more.

Also, avoid interruptions during a pleasant massage. Watching Sports center while getting a massage is less sensual. Silence the TV and focus on your partner's physique.

Good if your partner is keen on massaging you as well! Avoid expecting or demanding a massage. Make your partner happy.

Sensual massages don't always lead to sex. You and your lover can have a massage instead of becoming intimate.

THE END.

Printed in Great Britain
by Amazon